How to maintain good health and nutrition

27 things you should know about Natural Health and Nutrition

CHRIS WEILAND

Table of contents

Introduction

1. Limit your intake of sugary drinks.
Sugary drinks, such as sodas,

 fruit juices, and sweetened teas,
are the largest source of added sugar in
the American diet

Unfortunately,
multiple studies have found that sugar
sweetened beverages increase the risk of
heart

disease and diabetes even in those who do not have excess body fat .

Sugar-sweetened beverages are also particularly dangerous for children,
as they can contribute not

only to childhood obesity but also to conditions that usually do not develop until adulthood,
 such as

diabetes, high blood pressure, and liver disease
2. Consume nuts and seeds

Some people did not like nuts due to their high fat content.

Nuts and seeds, on the other hand, is aso heath seed.

They're high in protein, fiber, and vitamins and minerals .

Nuts may aid in weight loss and lower your risk of acquiring diabetes and heart disease

Chapter 1.

Furthermore,one major observational study found that a lack of nuts and seeds may be associated
with an increased risk of death.

3. Avoid highly processed foods.

Ultra-processed foods comprise elements that have been extensively altered from their natural state.

They frequently contain sugar, highy processed oil, sat, preservatives, artificial sweeteners, colors,

Here are several examples:

snacks and quick food
frozen dinners
cookies chips packaged
which means they are easily overeaten.

They also trigger reward related brain areas, which can lead
to excessive calorie consumption and weight gain.

Obesity, diabetes, heart disease, and other chronic

illnesses have all been linked to diets high in ultra-processed foods, according to research

4. Don't be afraid of coffee

Despite some disagreement, coffee has numerous health benefits.

Coffee is high in antioxidants, and some studies have connected it to onger life and a lower incidence

of diabetes, diseases, and a variety of other disorders .

Although 3-4 cups per day appears to be the most beneficial dosage, pregnant women should limit or

avoid it entirely because it has been associated to low birth weight

Chapter 2

However, coffee and other caffeine tea products should be consumed in moderation.

Taking
overdose can cause health problems such as sleeplessness and heart palpitations.

 Keep your coffee
consumption to fewer than 4 cups per day to stay safe and healthy

5. Consume fatty fish
Fish is a source of protein and healthful fat.

This is especially true for fatty fish like salmon, which contains
anti-inflammatory as well as other nutrients

Fish eaters find it so hard for them to develop heart disease, dementia, and inflammatory bowel disease.

6. Get enough rest
It is impossible to overestimate the value of getting enough quality sleep.

Sleep deprivation can increase insulin resistance,

affect appetite hormones, and impair physical and
mental function

Chapter 3

For more, lack of sleep is one of the most significant individual risk factors for weight gain and obesity.

People who don't get enough sleep tend to eat more fat, sugar, and calories, which can lead to
undesirable weight gain

7. Provide food for your gut bacteria

The bacteria in your gut, known as the gut microbiota, are extremely important for overall health.

A change in gut bacteria has been associated to a number of chronic disorders, including obesity and

a variety of digestive issues

Consuming fermented foods such as yogurt and sauerkraut,

taking probiotic supplements when
suggested, and eating enough of fiber are all
good strategies to boost gut health.

 Notably, fiber
functions as a prebiotic, or a source of food
for your gut bacteria

Chapter4.

8. Keep hydrated.
Hydration is a crucial but often overlooked health indicator.

Staying hydrated helps to ensure that your body is operating at peak efficiency and that your blood volume is enough

Water is the best way to maintain hydration because it contains no calories of sugar, or chemicals.

Although there is no defined quantity that everyone requires per day, aim to drink enough to satiate
your thirst.

9. Avoid eating burnt foods.

Meat can also be a healthy and nutritious part of your diet.

It contains a lot of protein and is a good

source of nutrients

However, issues may occur when meat is scorched or burnt.

This charing can result in the creation of hazardous chemicals, which may increase your risk of developing some cancers

When cooking meat avoid charring or burning it. Limit your diet of red and processed meats, such as

lunch meats and bacon, as these have been associated to an increased risk of colon cancer

Chapter 5

10. Avoid strong ights before going to bed.

When you are exposed to blue light wavelengths in the evening,
it may interfere with the production of
the sleep hormone melatonin

Wearing blue light blocking glasses especially if you use a computer or other digital screen for long

periods of time and avoiding digital devices for 30 minutes to an hour before going to bed are two

approaches to hep limit your blue light exposure
This can assist your body naturally manufacture melatonin as the evening continues,
allowing you to
sleep better.

11. If you are lacking in vitamin D, take it.
The majority of people do not get enough vitamin D.

While these widespread vitamin D deficiencies
are not immediately dangerous, maintaining adequate vitamin D levels can help to optimize your

health by improving bone strength, reducing depressive symptoms,

strengthening your immune
system, and lower your body from cancer .
Your vitamin D levels may be low if you do not spend a lot of time outside.
If you have access to it,
 it's a good idea to have your leves evaluated so you can rectify them with
vitamin D supplements if necessary.

Chapter 6

12. Consuming a variety of fruits and vegetables.

are high in prebiotic fiber, vitamins, mineras, and antioxidants, most of this things have powerful
health benefits.

People who consume more vegetables and fruits live longer and have a lower risk of heart disease,
obesity and other ailments..

13. Consume enough protein
Protein is essential for good health since it offers the raw resources your body requires to develop new
cells and tissues

Formore, this substance is critical for maintaining a healthy body weight.

A high protein diet could increase your metabolic rate (or calorie burn) while also making you feel full.

It may help lessen your desires and desire to nibble late at night

14. Get going!
Aerobic exercise, also known as cardio, is one of the most beneficial activities you can do for your
mental and physical health.

It's good at reducing fat in belly , which is dangerous fat that accumulates around in organs.
  Reduced abdominal fat may result in metabolic health

We should aim for at least 150 minutes of moderate intensity movement per week, according to the
Physical movement Guidelines for Americans

Chapter 7

15. Do not smoke or use drugs, and even drink only in moderation
Smoking, hazardous drugs , and alcohol can also have major consequences for your health.

Consider cutting back or quitting if you engage in any of these activities to help minimize your risk of
chronic diseases.

16. Use only extra virgin olive oil
One of the healthiest vegetable oils is extra virgin oive oil.

It contains heart-healthy monounsaturated fats as well as potent antioxidants with anti-inflammatory qualities

According to some data, those who eat extra virgin olive oil have a lower chance of dying from heart
attacks and strokes

17. Reduce your sugar intake.
Sugar is widely used in such foods and beverages.

Obesity, diabetes, and heart disease have all been
associated to a high intake

The Dietary Guidelines for Americans advocate limiting added sugar intake to less than 10% of daily
calories,
where as the Word Health Organisation recommends limiting added sugar intake to 5% or
fewer of daily calories for best health

Chapter 8

18. Limit your intake of processed carbohydrates.

Carbohydrates are not all made equal.

Refined carbohydrates have been heavily processed to remove fiber. Some people are lacking

nutrients which is not good,it might be harmful for your health,you must be careful with the food you
eat.

The majority of ultra processed foods are created with refined carbohydrates such as processed
corn, white flour and added sugars.

A diet high in refined carbohydrates has been associated to overeating, weight gain, and chronic
diseases such as diabetes and heart disease

19. Lift weights.

Strength and resistance training are two of the most effective types of workouts for building muscle
and improving body composition
.

It may aso result in significant improvements in metabolic health, such as increased insulin sensitivity,

which means your blood sugar levels are simper to maintain, and increases in metabolic rate, or how
many calories you burn at rest
If you don't have weights,

you can produce resistance using your own bodyweight or resistance
bands and receive a comparable workout with many of the same advantages.
Resistance exercise should be done twice a week, according to the Physical Activity Guidelines for
Americans.

Chapter 9

20. Work out using weights.

Strength and resistance training are two of the most effective types of workouts for muscle gain and
body composition improvement.

It may also lead to major gains in metabolic health, such as greater insulin sensitivity, which means

your blood sugar levels are easier to control, and increases in metabolic rate, or how many calories
you burn at rest

If you don't have weights, you can get a comparable workout with many of the same benefits by using

your own bodyweight or resistance bands.

According to the Physical Activity Guidelines for Americans resistance training should be done twice a
week

21. Make use of herbs and spices
More than ever before,

we have access herbs and spices. They not only add favor but may
also have some health advantages .

Ginger and turmeric, for example, offer powerful anti inflammatory and antioxidant properties that
may benefit your general health

You should been using variety of herbs and spices in your diet because of their great potential health
benefits.

Chapter 10

22. Take care of your social contacts.
Social ties – with friends, family, and loved ones — are critical not only for your mental health but also
for your physical health.

Studies reveal that persons who have close friends and family live substantially longer lives than those
who do not

23. Track your food intake on a regular basis.

Some people may benefit from measuring their food and using a nutrition tracker to determine how
many calories they consume

Tracking can also reveal information about your protein, fiber, and
vitamin intake.

While tracking may help some people manage their weight, there is evidence that it can also

contribute to disordered eating
Before implementing this technique consult with your doctor.

24. Remove extra tummy fat
Excess abdominal fat, also known as visceral fat,

is a form of fat distribution that has been associated
to an elevated risk of cardiometabolic disorders such as diabetes and heart disease

As a result, your size and waist-to hip ratio may be far more accurate than your weight.

Reducing refined carbs, increasing protein and fiber consumption, and lowering stress (which can
lower cortisol,

a stress hormone that causes abdominal fat
deposition) are all measures that may
help you reduce belly fat

Chapter 11

25. Avoid rigid diets.

Indeed, previous dieting is one of the best predictors of future weight gain

This is due to the fact that excessively restrictive diets lower your metabolic rate, or the quantity of
calories you burn,

making it more difficult to lose weight.
 At the same time, they change your hunger and satiety hormones,
   making you hungrier and potentially leading to intense food cravings for meals heavy in fat, calories, and sugar

This is a recipe for rebound weight gain sometimes known as "yoyo" dieting.

Weight loss should occur as you move to whoe, healthy foods which are inherently more satisfying and have less calories than processed items

26. Consume entire eggs
Despite the continual debate regarding eggs and health, it is a fallacy that eggs are unhealthy due to
their high cholesterol level.

 According to research, they have no effect on blood cholesterol in the
majority of people and are an excellent source of protein and nutrients

For more, a study of 263938 participants revealed no link between egg consumption and the
incidence of heart disease

Conclusion

27. Practice meditation
Stress is detrimental to your health. It can
an impact on your blood sugar levels, food
choices, illness,

weight, fat distribution, and other factors.
As a result, it's critical to identify
appropriate ways to handle
stress

Meditation is one such method, and there is
some scientific evidence to back up its use
for stress
management and health improvement

Researchers discovered that meditation
helped lower LDL (bad) cholesterol and
inflammation in one
trial including 48 participants with high
blood pressure type 2 diabetes, or both.

Furthermore,

meditation group participants reported better mental and physical wellness

A few simple strategies can help you improve your eating habits and overall health.

Likewise, if you want to live a better life, don't just focus on eating things you don't know how it been
preserve....

Exercise, seep, and social interactions are also essential.

With the evidence-based advice provided above,
 it is simple to implement tiny adjustments that can
have a significant influence on your overall health.